Aerobic
Dancing
a Step at a Time

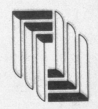

Aerobic
Dancing
a Step at a Time

Phyllis Sawyer and Pat Thornton

Contemporary Books, Inc.
Chicago

Library of Congress Cataloging in Publication Data

Sawyer, Phyllis.
    Aerobic dancing a step at a time.

    Includes index.
    1. Aerobic exercises.   2. Dancing.   I. Thornton,
Pat.   II. Title.
RA781.15.S28   1981   613.7′1   81-65176
ISBN 0-8092-5958-3 (pbk.)   AACR2

Photographs: Pat Thornton
              Ansgar Johnson

*This book is dedicated to Jim Everett,
physical director of the Boise Family
YMCA. There is no one more sincere in his
efforts to help people of all ages gain better
self-images than Jim. He has truly been an
inspiration to both of us.*

Contents

Preface   *ix*

1. Purpose   *1*

2. The Basics   *4*

3. Aerobic Dance   *8*

4. Clothing   *11*

5. Getting Started   *16*

6. Dos, Don'ts, and Cautions   *24*

7. Language   *28*

8. Warming Up   *62*

9. Aerobic Dance Routines   *72*

10. Cool-Downs   *86*

Index   *97*

Preface

Phyllis Sawyer and I have spent many of our waking hours involved in some form of physical exercise. We were physical education majors in college when we learned the joys of sharing our knowledge by teaching others to enjoy sports and by sharing the good feeling that comes with fitness.

Although we grew up in different parts of the country, we met at the Boise, Idaho, Family YMCA, where both of us teach fitness classes. Phyllis leads aerobic dance, while I am involved in the "Run for Your Life" program.

This book is a natural for both of us because we are concerned about the sudden 'health craze' that often has unqualified people selling fitness. We feel that such activity results in many people either getting hurt, ripped off, or both.

As Phyllis says: "Many of these people aren't teaching fitness; they're making a quick buck. As a result, a lot of people are suffering. I think, with the interest in this relatively new 'sport' of aerobic dance, there are a lot of 'dance' instructors who are performing artists rather than instructors. They seem to think they are there to put on a show demonstrating the degree of difficulty they can achieve."

Our aim in writing this book is to help people learn about potential problem areas of their bodies, such as the cardiovascular system, and to begin correctly as they try to improve both their physical health and their fitness level.

Pat Thornton

Aerobic
Dancing
a Step at a Time

1
Purpose

Welcome to the world of feeling good! You are about to embark on a program that will improve your physical and mental image, not only for today, but for years to come as well.

Welcome to the world of aerobics! Don't let that word "aerobics" stop you. It simply means the use of air: oxygen.

Aerobic exercise is anything that requires the body to demand more than normal amounts of oxygen for a prolonged period of time. Some forms of aerobic exercise are: fast walking, jogging, running, swimming, bicycling, jumping rope. In other words, any exercise that gets your heart rate up and uses increased oxygen levels through breathing is an aerobic exercise.

Increased oxygen levels lead to physical fitness, an acknowledged important contribution to general health. Exercise as a preventative has few equals. Almost all forms of aerobic exercise are inexpensive and practical. Most of all, they have proven to be highly effective in combating many health problems ranging from a simple backache to America's leading killer: coronary heart disease.

There is an old saying that "Man does not die; he kills himself." From all evidence based on the average American's sedentary lifestyle and eating habits, that statement is truer today than ever before. More people are killing themselves with alcohol and cigarettes, wrong foods, excess weight, and lack of exercise than ever died from medieval diseases. That is why Dr. Richard Keelor, program director for the President's Council on Physical Fitness, sometimes refers to heart disease and lung cancer as "diseases of choice."

Statistics reported by the President's Council on Physical Fitness show that 95 percent of the people of America are out of shape. Most Americans don't exercise at all, except to walk to the refrigerator and to the TV set to switch channels. Studies show that of those Americans who do participate in some form of physical activity, many either don't have the right approach to exercise or don't exercise properly. Walking across the street to the neighbor's for a cup of coffee or a beer once a week is not exercise.

Did you know that coronary heart disease accounts for approximately four out of ten deaths? When you take into account other blood circulation problems, such as stroke and high blood pressure, every second death in the United States is of cardiovascular origin. Today, about one out of every ten deaths before the age of 35 is blamed on some form of heart disease.

Thomas K. Cureton, of the Physical Fitness Laboratory at the University of Illinois, has come up with some startling facts: The average American young man has a middle-aged body, and he cannot run a city block, or climb a flight of stairs without becoming out of breath. Cureton says that a man in his twenties today has the capacity that a man is expected to have in his forties. In this area, women are becoming more and more like their male counterparts.

The obvious way to combat these startling statistics is to become involved in a proper fitness program of aerobic exercise. Aerobic exercises strengthen the cardiovascular system and make it a more efficient machine when it is resting, working, sleeping, and, of course, exercising.

What we're talking about is conditioning of the cardiovascular pulmonary system, which involves the heart, lungs, and blood vessels. Without that conditioning, you will never be physically fit. Improvement to, or conditioning of, the cardiovascular pulmonary system comes only when the work load is greater than that to which the individual is accustomed. Achieving high levels of physical working capacity can only be accomplished by endurance work of sufficient intensity and duration to challenge the circulorespiratory systems.

Therefore, the purpose of aerobic exercise, and, in this case, aerobic dance, is to increase the working capacity of the cardiovascular pulmonary system. That spells f-i-t-n-e-s-s. And fitness results in feeling good mentally as well as physically, giving yourself a lift and a whole new outlook on life.

2
The Basics

As we've said, aerobic exercise is anything that requires the body to demand more than normal amounts of oxygen for a prolonged period of time. Any exercise that gets your heart rate up and uses increased oxygen levels through breathing is an aerobic exercise.

Do not, however, be drawn into an anaerobic exercise thinking that just because your heart beat goes up you are doing aerobics. An anaerobic is a start-and-stop sport, such as gymnastics, skiing, the 100-yard dash, tennis, golf. These are all fine forms of exercise, and they do increase your skill, but the oxygen is cut short. An anaerobic exercise is like a vacation—it doesn't last long enough.

Whatever aerobic activity you choose, be sure to allow enough time in your schedule to maintain an intensity level of sufficient duration. Do not, for example, jump rope for three minutes and think you've done your aerobics for the day. Three minutes is just a good start.

Ideally, your aerobic activity should continue non-stop anywhere for a minimum of 12 minutes to 20 minutes, or longer. The levels of intensity and of duration are usually not achieved until the body has developed sufficient heat from within to bring about sweating.

Let us stop for a minute and say a few words about "sweat." This is not a dirty word. Sweat is a human body function. It is very natural and is the body's way of cooling itself. Expect to sweat. Expect your clothes to become damp and your hair to stick to the back of your neck, and don't be embarrassed about it.

Back to aerobics. The basic philosophy behind aerobic exercise is that it is the only real kind of exercise for fitness.

What, you may ask, is fitness? It is, indeed, very hard to define because fitness involves a number of factors. Clayton R. Myers, in his *The Official YMCA Physical Fitness Handbook*, says, "Technically, it is a measure of the body's strength, endurance, and flexibility. In a more personal sense, it is the capacity to do hard work for a *continuous period of time without diminishing efficiency.* It is a condition that involves good coordination of the body, mind, and spirit."

Another description we came across calls fitness a "dynamic, positive thing—not merely the absence of disease. There are many elements of physical fitness such as endurance, balance, power, strength, flexibility, and agility. But in the final analysis, the real test of fitness is intuitive. It is how you feel. How you feel in the morning; how you feel about playing with the children after work or going out with friends at night."

The benefits of being fit are many. There is an increased energy and stamina level. There is confidence and a positive feeling toward yourself that results from better general health. There is the ability to better handle life's stresses and tensions. Usually, there is a weight loss, or, at least, an inches loss. An increased natural selectivity in the types of foods eaten results in a better nutritional status.

Other benefits include an improvement in sleep and rest; the ability to participate in many types of both recreational and leisure activities; a reduction in cigarette smoking; a reduction in total food intake; and, most of all, the development of an exercise habit that continues throughout life.

From a personal point of view, Phyllis looks at the benefits of fitness this way: "Of course there is a weight loss, inch loss, body fat loss. Exercise has been proven to improve your heart rate, and slow it down. It lowers your blood pressure; improves your flexibility and coordination; helps you deal with daily stress; gives you a little more energy than you might have.

"How does it deal, or help deal, with stress? I suppose because the blood exchange within the body is more efficient, the body itself becomes a better user of oxygen. The body becomes a more efficient user of oxygen, because it is a better working machine.

"I know aerobic exercise takes away stress. I remember when I was running (and I had very small children at the time), people used to say to me, 'Why do you do that?' And I would answer, 'When I run in the morning, I don't have to take a tranquilizer in the afternoon.' It was something I could feel; something I could understand.

"I ran before jogging was in vogue, and I didn't understand the philosophy behind it. I didn't understand that doing an aerobic exercise was improving my heart rate. I didn't know about these things. Now that I do know what aerobics can do, I personally know that philosophy to be true.

"Why was I active in aerobic exercise if I didn't know the physiological reasons behind it? I did it because it made me feel good. It made it easier for me to handle my day-to-day living."

Coping and feeling good are, of course, welcome benefits, you may say, but, why is there a relationship between being fit and the reduction of chances of a heart attack? Why is there a relationship between fitness and improvement of the chances of survival of a heart attack?

There are six widely accepted reasons:

(1) Development of a stronger and more efficient heart muscle
(2) Reduced blood pressure both during exercise and at rest

(3) Reduced heart rate both during exercise and at rest
(4) Lowered levels of blood cholesterol and triglycerides
(5) A decrease in the susceptibility of the heart-to-rhythm disturbances
(6) Development of collateral circulation

Age is a very important factor in people's minds when considering whether to become involved in an exercise program. It's not that age is limiting, but the fact that many adults think of themselves as being "too old" when, actually, the opposite is true: The need for exercise increases with age.

Do you know when the human body reaches physiological middle age? It is not the magic age of 40, as many believe. Actually, 26 is the age at which the body begins to decline. Much of that decline is attributed to lack of use. The body starts to break down and continues to do so until it is almost useless. Therefore, the only time that age becomes a restriction and bothers you is when you are not exercising regularly. If you are in a regular fitness routine, age is no factor.

So: "Use it or lose it."

3
Aerobic Dance

Through long years of experience and participation, we have learned that aerobic exercise is really the only exercise for fitness. Aerobic dance is not the only kind of beneficial aerobic exercise, but it certainly is an excellent form of it. Other good forms of aerobics include: jogging, running, jumping rope, fast bicycling, fast walking.

So what form is best? We're not going to single out any one kind. Unless you particularly enjoy a certain exercise, you will probably become bored in time, and lose interest. What you should be looking for is something you can do for a lifetime, not just a five-week or a six-week class.

Thus, rather than say aerobic dance is the only way to become fit for a lifetime, we'd rather tell you to participate in a combination of exercises. For example, you can do aerobic dance two or three times a week; run or jog a few mornings each week; and ride your bicycle on Sunday. Then you will have a well-rounded aerobic exercise program.

But, for the time being, we'll settle for your participation in an aerobic exercise three times a week. That does not mean working three consecutive days, such as Monday, Tuesday, Wednesday, and laying off the next four. The best program to begin with is to work alternate days, such as Monday, Wednesday, Friday. Later, as you begin feeling better and more fit, your body will ask for more of a work load and you will, naturally and voluntarily, increase your participation. Expect to feel a positive change in about three weeks' time.

Remember, to improve your aerobic fitness, you need to work; you need to have your heart rate up to its working level anywhere from 12 to 20 minutes. So, we would suggest you set aside 30 to 40 minutes for exercise. You warm up a little; then go into the aerobic part; and, finally, spend time cooling down and stretching. In all, that will take 30 to 40 or 45 minutes. Count on using that much time. Do not skimp in any of the three areas, because each is of vital importance.

As we've said before, an aerobic exercise is one that requires the body to demand more than normal amounts of oxygen for a prolonged period of time. One type exercise that fits the description perfectly is aerobic dance.

We are often asked to define aerobic dance. It has been described as choreographed jogging. Or, running to music. Or, exercising to rhythm. It is all of these; it really is not dance.

Phyllis, who has been doing and teaching aerobic dance long before the activity had a name, says she created the routines in this book by listening to music then adding motions to match the tempo. Most of them have some kind of stretching movement or strengthening movement in them. They are not "dance routines." They are fitness routines set to music. If a dancer were to walk into an aerobic dance class, she would shake her head and say, "This is not really dance." She would be right. It is not dance; it is movement to music for fitness.

Anyone can do aerobic dance. Fat people can do it, thin people, young people, old people. Why? Because the whole thing is based on common sense. If you are very much out of shape, very heavy, then you are going to have to move slowly. Out-of-shape people cannot kick as high, or hold their arms up in the air as well as someone who is fit; but they can still do the routines. They can still begin to tone the muscles. They can still begin to lose the body fat. They will probably lose weight faster than someone who is not as heavy, because they have more fat to burn. That's what aerobics does: it gets rid of excess fat in the body. If you eat sensibly and become involved in an aerobics program, you can expect to look and feel better fast.

Chances are that if you are not really overweight, you may initially find a weight gain as far as the scales are concerned. The reason is that, as you become fit, the fat in your body is being replaced by muscle fiber and muscle weighs more than fat. Nevertheless, if you do find an initial weight gain on the scales, at the same time you will probably start seeing an inch loss because the muscle tone is improving and the fat is being lost.

Incidentally, aerobic dance is an excellent form of exercise for both women and men. This is why we stress that aerobic dance is not really dance. There are some programs based on a lot of ballet, and the majority of men are not interested in those. However, we prefer to think of our program as an aerobic activities-type class in which there is movement to rhythm and there is dance in it, but anyone can learn it.

Several men have joined the aerobic dance class at the Boise Y, and they don't have any more problem catching on to the routines than the women. It just takes a little time. Before long, the male students are having just as much fun and enjoying all of the benefits of better health and well-being.

4
Clothing

There is much that can be said about what to wear. Basically, the best advice is keep it simple, keep it comfortable and keep it loose. Aerobic dance, like most other athletic activities, is not a fashion show and does not require the "latest" in colors and styles. You can wear leotards and bodysuits, shorts and teeshirts, or sweatpants and sweatshirts.

Personal opinion on fabrics themselves varies widely. However, we feel whatever you wear should be made of a breathable material. Cotton is the best because it not only allows the skin to breathe but, more importantly, the fabric absorbs body moisture.

Some of the newer man-made materials do offer advantages in stretchability and a few of them do breathe. However, it is obvious that most of the synthetics do not breathe as well as cotton, because you can often see blotches of perspiration in areas of the body, such as armpits, tummy, and the small of the back. Another disadvantage of some synthetics is permanent sweat-stains.

If the area in which you are exercising is cool, layering of clothing is a good idea. Attention should be paid to legs, in particular, and, depending upon the individual, to the upper torso, too. Sweatpants and shirts or a warm-up suit worn over less bulky clothing, such as teeshirts or bodysuits, is a good idea to begin. Then, as your body temperature reaches working level, strip off the outer layer, and continue the routines wearing the lighter clothes. Remember, as a rule of thumb, if the temperature was cool enough when you started to warrant layering, you will want to add the other clothes again as you begin your cool-downs.

For women, a supportive bra is of prime importance and mandatory for some. From experience, we have learned that bras used for dress and bras used for sport are vastly different in construction, and "never the twain shall meet." In other words, that soft, pretty, lacy bra women wear under a sheer blouse is of no value during physical activity.

A sport bra should be made of firm material, somewhat elastic in nature. You need support, but you also need freedom of movement. We have had good experience with the brand Jogbra, a sport bra developed by two women runners who saw the need for better support. The bra can be found at most sporting goods stores.

Men will want to wear a jockstrap or similar undergarment, not only for support, but for comfort as well.

Now, let's talk about shoes. Exercising barefoot should be discouraged. Your feet need protection, and the rest of your body needs the support provided by good shoes. Good shoes are the key not only to comfort, but also to injury prevention. They will help prevent foot problems and shin splints, to say nothing of the problems of arch and heel, leg and knee, and even of the back.

When buying shoes, expect to pay at least $25 or more for a good pair. Anything priced less, including "specials" offered at discount stores, is probably inferior and could result in both injury and discomfort. Although that initial $25 or more seems expensive on the surface, consider that it is the only cash outlay you will have to make, because everything else can come out of your drawer, or your kids' drawers.

The shoes you select should be highly supportive, with a well-cushioned sole for shock absorption. They should be flexible, light in weight, durable, and offer good stability and motion control. They should have bottoms that give good traction.

The shoe you should look for is one that fits all of these criteria. It may, or may not, be a running and/or jogging shoe. A person who is an avid tennis player, for example, may find everything he wants in a tennis shoe. You may find a volleyball shoe best fits your needs, or a basketball shoe. Avoid any shoe with cleats. Football, soccer, rugby shoes will not meet your requirements, because they will not pass the stability test on a non-grassy surface.

When shopping for shoes, don't be in a rush. Take the time to give your prospective shoes a fair test, and go to a store where the clerks don't mind your trying shoes and walking around a bit. Also, don't be swayed by what your neighbor says is the best, or what the clerk claims is today's most popular shoe. What's right for someone else may be totally wrong for you. There is only one way to select a shoe: by how it feels on your foot.

"If the shoe fits, wear it!" How can you be sure if the fit is right? There are several tests. Begin by wearing the socks, pantyhose, footlets or whatever you will usually wear between skin and shoe because the fit is very important. The shoes should be snug, but not tight in width, and there should be plenty of toe room. Shoes that are too big or too small will cause blisters; shoes that are too small will limit circulation.

Because in aerobic dance the tendency is to work toward the front of the foot, you will probably require more length than you would in a walking shoe. So basically, with the laces untied and your toes touching the front, if you can slip a finger behind your heel (Figure 1), you have a good fit.

You can also test for size by standing on a slant (Figure 2). If your foot slides forward from the heel, consider a smaller

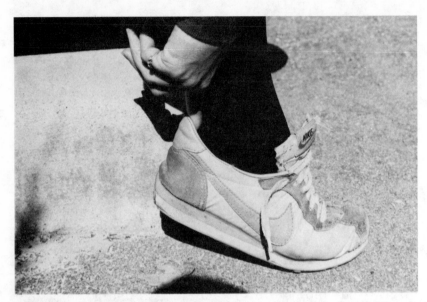

Figure 1. Finger behind heel

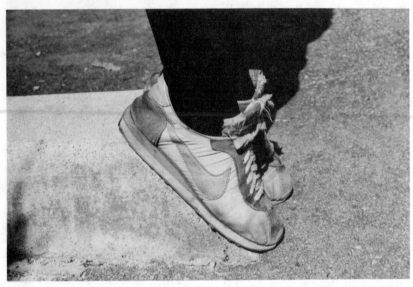

Figure 2. Stand on a slant

size. Or, lace up the shoes and try to work your heel up and down inside while holding the outside firm (Figure 3). If you can move the heel, a smaller size is in order.

Remember the importance of good, well-fitting shoes. Bargain shoes are not necessarily bargains in the long run.

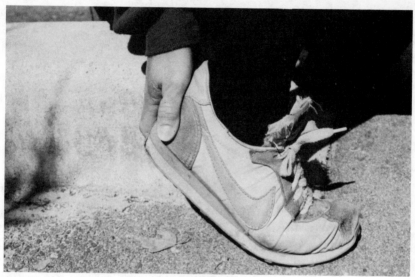

Figure 3. Hold the heel

5
Getting Started

Phyllis got started in aerobic dance simply because she has always enjoyed music and dancing. In the wintertime when her children were small, she recalls spending "a lot of mornings of my life dancing around the house. For me it was a very simple thing to put on the records and to do some routines and do them consistently. The kids did them, too, following my lead. We marched around the house to music and did all kinds of activities to rhythm."

Phyllis is probably unique in her approach to exercise and her willingness to start off on her own. For a lot of people an exercise program like aerobic dance is a social experience. For that reason, we suggest participation might be something you should do with a friend. If you can make it a family experience, that's all the better. Aerobics is something that all ages can do. If everyone doesn't know a particular routine, it doesn't matter because learning comes with time. Aerobic dance is simply moving to the music as you get your heart beat up to a working rate and keep it up there for 12 to 20 minutes.

Do you know what your pulse rate is? Or how to take it? There are several places on the body where the pulse is easy to find. The most common and preferred spot is the radial artery, on the thumbside of your wrist (Figure 4). Another, and often easier, place is found by lightly placing the second finger at your throat on either side of your voice box on the carotid artery (Figure 5).

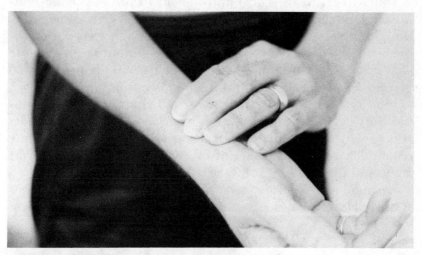

Figure 4. Pulse at radial artery

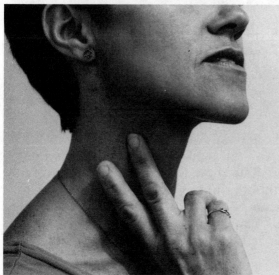

Figure 5. Pulse at carotid artery

When taking your pulse, count for ten seconds and multiply that number by six. The total is your heart rate for one minute.

We'll be using two terms referring to specific heart rates: Resting Heart Rate and Target Heart Rate. To find out the Resting Heart Rate, take your pulse when the heart is at rest. Like right now, as you read this book.

You will recall we said improvement in physical conditioning and in the cardiovascular pulmonary system comes only through aerobic exercise. Achievement in high levels of physical working capacity comes only by endurance work, while your heart is beating at 80 percent of its maximum. That 80 percent figure is called your Target or Working Heart Rate.

Here is a formula the YMCA uses to establish your individual Target Heart Rate: begin with the figure 220 and subtract your age. Then subtract your Resting Heart Rate from the remainder. Multiply the result by .80. Add your Resting Heart Rate, and the total is your Target Heart Rate.

As an example, let's say you are 40 years old and your Resting Heart Rate is 70:

$$
\begin{array}{r}
220 \\
-\underline{\quad 40}\ \text{(your age)} \\
180 \\
-\underline{\quad 70}\ \text{(your Resting Heart Rate)} \\
110 \\
\times\ \underline{\ .80} \\
88 \\
+\underline{\quad 70}\ \text{(your Resting Heart Rate)} \\
158
\end{array}
$$

So, if you are 40 years old and your Resting Heart Rate is 70, your Target Heart Rate should reach 158 beats per minute for from 12 to 20 minutes or longer during the aerobic portion of your exercise program.

It is important that you monitor your heart frequently. We suggest you take your pulse at the end of each dance routine.

Another method of keeping tabs on your heart is the Talk Test. This is a very good guideline. If you cannot talk, if you cannot carry on a conversation, while you are doing an aerobic exercise, you are working too hard.

In addition to good shoes, a clock or watch that has a sweep second hand, and either a record player or tape recorder on which to play the music, there is one other item we suggest you have: a cobra (Figure 6).

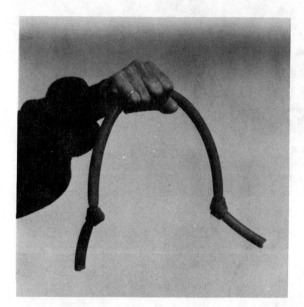

Figure 6. Cobra

For want of a better name, that's what they are called at the Y. They are pieces of surgical tubing, which is readily available at hospital or medical supply stores. You will want a piece about 18 inches in length with a knot tied in both ends. The cobra's main purpose is upper arm toning, not necessarily strength or muscle development, but toning the muscles. It seems to do a lot for both the bicep and the tricep.

To use a cobra, hold the tubing with your fists against each knot (Figure 7). Pull it as far as you can without a lot of strain, then release it slowly. Don't let it snap back; keep a little tension in there. Normally, when you start working with a cobra you can feel it, probably the most through your upper arms. Through continued use, you will find the tension less and less. At that point, you can shorten up on the tube, moving your hands a little closer together.

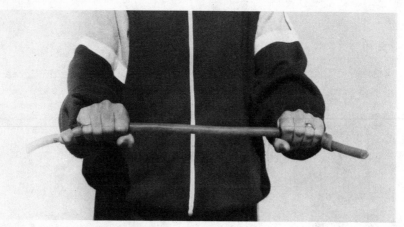

Figure 7. Basic cobra position

While standing, start by stretching the cobra in front of you at chest level. Then stretch it from your forehead (Figure 8), at your hips, up over your head with arms stretched straight up, at your navel, straight out from your shoulder (Figure 9), behind your neck (Figure 10).

There's one other thing to do with a cobra. Standing straight with arms in front at waist level, stretch the cobra taut. Keeping it taut, raise your arms over your head, turn your upper body to the left and bend from the waist (Figure 11). When you reach the floor, relax the tube slowly and curl your body up to the standing position. Repeat, turning to the right, then again down the center.

As we said, the cobra is a very good way to tone and strengthen muscles. Another good method is with push-ups.

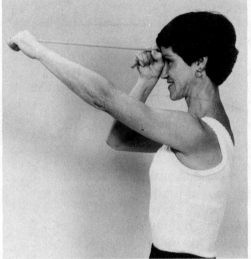

Figure 8. Cobra stretched
from forehead

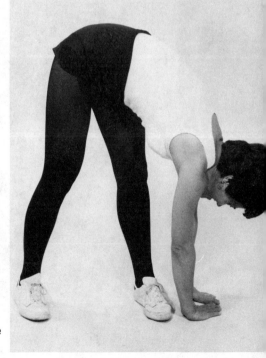

Figure 9. Cobra stretched
from shoulder

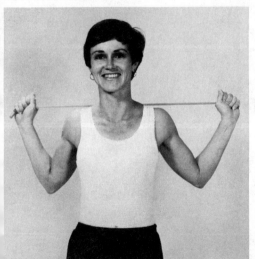

Figure 10. Cobra stretched
behind neck

Figure 11. Bend left to the
floor

We agree, push-ups are a drag, but they are also excellent conditioners and, if done properly, are not that difficult. There is a tendency to think of push-ups as being all arms. Arms are, of course, important, but what you are really developing and strengthening are the abdominal or stomach muscles. It's the abdominals that keep your body straight during a push-up. Besides, push-ups are something where results are readily evident—today, you can do five; tomorrow, you may be able to do seven.

Here are some things to remember about push-ups. The proper position is very important. Your hands should be in a diamond-shape (Figure 12) with your thumbs placed approximately under your nipples. You may have to adjust your hands in or out a little, depending upon the width of your shoulders and the length of your arms, but do start with this guideline for distance between your hands.

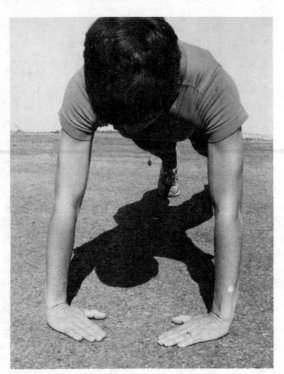

Figure 12. Push-up hand position

Beginners should never do push-ups from the toes. Start out on your knees with your feet bent up (Figure 13). This position takes the strain off your back as you build up the abdominals to hold your body straight. So start doing push-ups from your knees until they are easy and your abdominals strong; then you can move down to your toes (Figure 14).

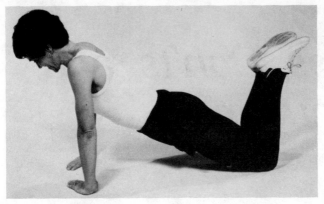

Figure 13. Bent-knee push-up

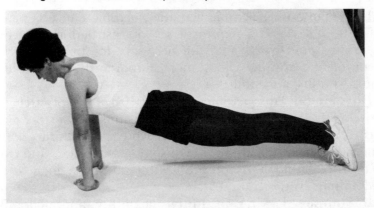

Figure 14. Push-up fully extended from the toes

The routines in this book are not difficult and most are fairly repetitious and, therefore, are not hard to learn to do in your own living room. So, gather the family and the neighbors around, check the dos and don'ts, learn the language or descriptions of steps and you are ready to begin.

6
Dos, Don'ts, and Cautions

Like many other aerobic activities, aerobic dance is neither difficult, nor does it require a lot of instruction. However, there are some basics that are necessary for proper development of the routines and, more importantly, for avoiding pains, sprains, and strains.

Do start out any aerobic exercise with a lot of stretching movements. You have to look at each and be sensible about them. You have to know whether you can get into a full-length push-up position, for instance, and flex your midsection to the floor. If you are flexible and have good, strong abdominals, you can do that.

If you are lacking in initial flexibility and abdominal strength, you cannot do a full-length push-up and you *do* have to work up to it slowly. If you go into aerobic dance hard, it's just like anything else: you will get hurt, and you're likely to wash out of the program. If you *do* go into the exercises gradually, you are more likely to enjoy the experience.

Aerobic dance routines are not difficult or hard to learn, but they can be strenuous, and that's where you have to be your own judge. You *do* have to slow down when you reach a point where the routine is too hard for you.

While going through the dance numbers, *do not* work up on your toes. You should try to work on the balls of your feet or lower, if you can. When you get up on your toes, the result is a tightening of the muscles in your calves and, chances are, in the beginning, you will get a charley horse or some other kind of cramp in your calf.

After you are finished with your exercises, be sure to stretch out those calves. That is a very important part of the program—you *do* need to stretch out. There is a natural tendency in aerobic dance to shorten the calf muscles, just as there is in running, so the stretching, the cool-down part, is very important.

Another thing to remember is that any time you are in a standing position and are bending down, *do not* do it with a straight back. You should never bend from the waist with your back straight. Instead, tuck your chin into your neck and curl down to the floor (Figures 15A–15C).

Figure 15A. Tuck your chin into your neck and curl down to the floor

Figure 15B. Bend at waist and keep your chin tucked in

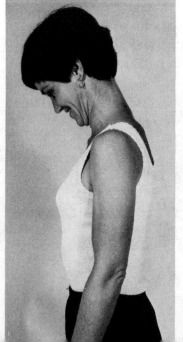

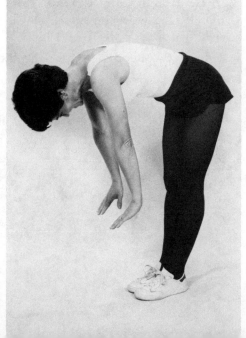

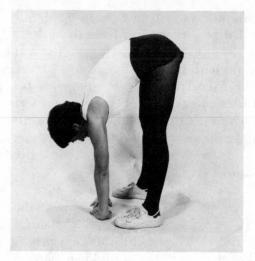

Figure 15C. All the way down to the floor

When you come back up, *do* exactly the same thing: round your back and curl up, tucking your chin into your neck.

A doctor compared bending from the waist with a straight back to holding a 12-pound ball on the end of a stick. It is very difficult to raise and lower that 12-pound ball. He said that is exactly what you do every time you go up and down with a straight back; your head is heavy. So *do* curl down and *do* curl back up. That way you take the strain off your back.

The same thing applies when you are doing a sit-up. *Do* use the same curling principle—tuck your chin into your neck, round your back and come up (Figures 16A and 16B). Then lead with the small of your back as you go down. Also, when doing a sit-up, *do* bend your knees instead of keeping

Figure 16A. Bent-knee sit-up. Do the curling principle.

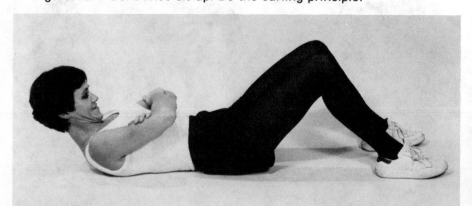

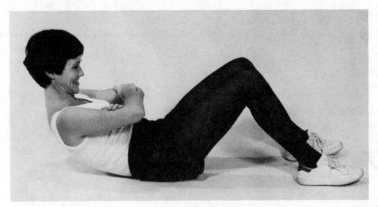

Figure 16B. Tuck your chin into your neck, round your back, and come up

your legs flat on the floor. The bent-knee relieves the strain on your lower back.

Still avoiding back strain, any time you do an exercise lying on your back with your legs off the floor—as in scissoring your legs open and close or straddling your legs—you *do* need to raise your head off the floor, too. Lifting the head takes the strain off your lower back.

In doing floor exercises, you should place your hands near the small of your back so you can tell if your back arches. If your back does arch off the floor, it is a sign your abdominal muscles are not strong enough yet to work lower. So *do* raise your legs higher until your back does not arch. As you become more fit, you can lower your legs gradually until your back stays down. Incidentally, in even the most fit people, the back will arch a little bit, but if you try it, you can tell the difference; one is a strain, one is not a strain.

Anytime you stretch into any kind of a lunge position, reach for the floor, reach to the side, or just reach, stretch and hold; *do not* bounce back and forth, up and down. Bouncing will not stretch your muscle, but it might tear the muscle and cause formation of scar tissue, which means you will never be able to stretch as far. The best way to stretch muscles is to go as far as you can, hold the position for a few seconds, then relax.

And *do* re-read what we said in Chapter 5 about push-ups. Position is very important.

7
Language

Every activity has its own language. Naturally, aerobic dance does, too, although these same terms apply to and are used in other exercise forms. Many of them will be familiar to you, while others will require an explanation or definition.

There are many other movements, but the terminology defined here is confined to that used in the routines within this book.

Bicycle: This exercise is done in different positions. The basic posture is sitting on the floor with your upper body leaning back resting on bent arms. Your legs are extended while moving in a circular motion similar to that of riding a bicycle.

Bicycle to Left: Assume the basic bicycle position with the upper body comfortably supported. Roll to the left hip. In that position, move your legs in the basic bicycle motion.

Bicycle to Right: Assume the basic bicycle position with your upper body comfortably supported. Roll to the right hip. In that position, move your legs in the basic bicycle motion.

Straddle: Stand with legs approximately shoulder-width apart (Figure 17).

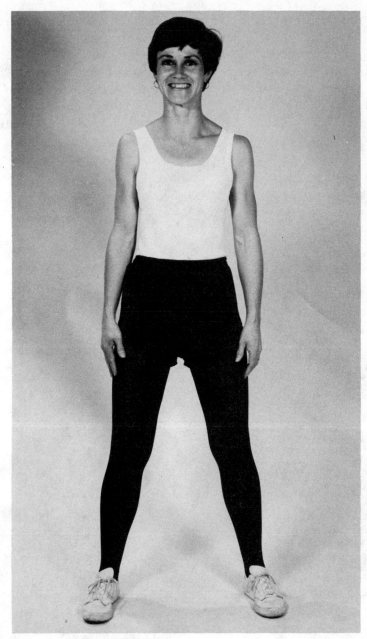

Figure 17. Straddle jump

Straddle Jump: This is a two-movement action. Stand with legs together; then jump to land with legs in a straddle position. Jump back to starting position.

Jumping Jack: This is a two-movement action. Start with legs together and arms at sides. Jump to straddle position as arms move upward (Figures 18A–18C) and touch overhead (Figure 18D). Jump back to starting position with arms returning to sides (Figure 18E).

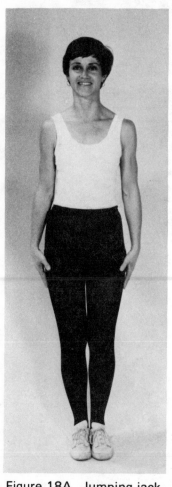

Figure 18A. Jumping jack

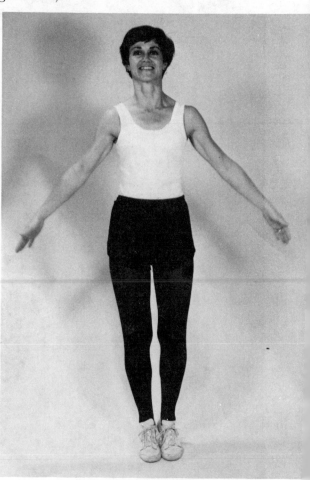

Figure 18B. Raise arms

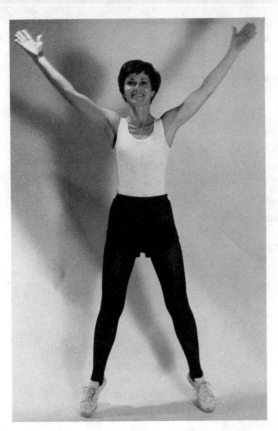

Figure 18C. Jump to straddle position

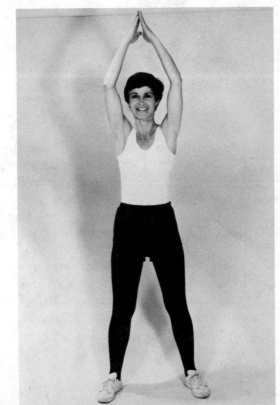

Figure 18D. Touch hands over head

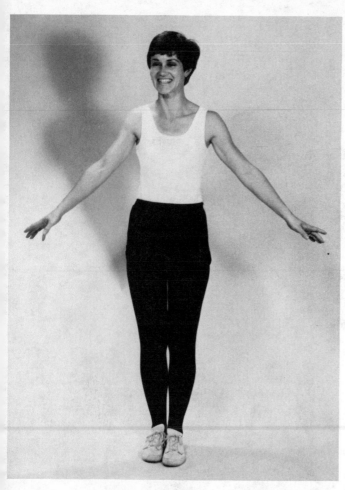

Figure 18E. Lower arms as you jump back to starting position

Squat: With legs in straddle position, lower body toward the floor. Be sure to keep your back straight and your heels on the floor. Return to straddle position (Figure 19).

Reach Right: Begin with arms down at the sides and in front of the body. Swing arms together up and toward the right until both are reaching straight. Turn body slightly toward the right with the swinging motion (Figure 20).

Reach Left: Begin with arms down at the sides and in front of the body. Swing arms together up and toward the left until both are reaching straight. Turn body slightly toward the left with the swinging motion.

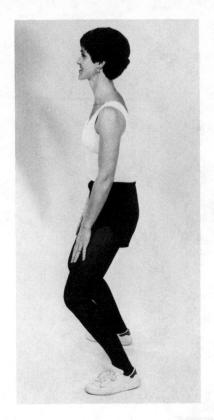

Figure 19. Squat

Figure 20. Reach
right

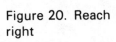

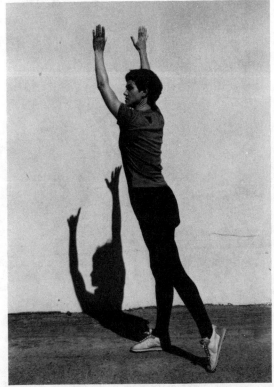

Reach Up: Begin with both arms down at the sides and in front of the body. Swing arms together up until both are reaching straight up. Lift your chin up with the movement of the arms. (Figure 21).

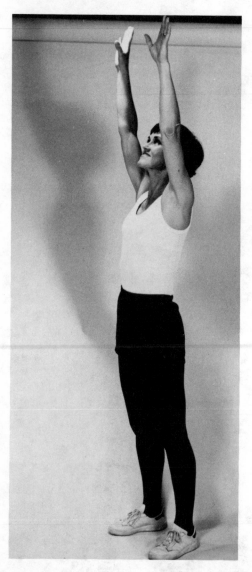

Figure 21. Reach up

Jog Circle: Jog while turning in a small circle (Figures 22A–22E).

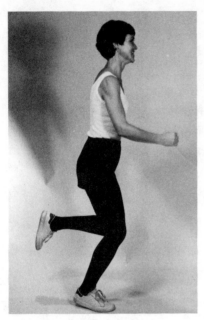

Figure 22A. Jog in a circle

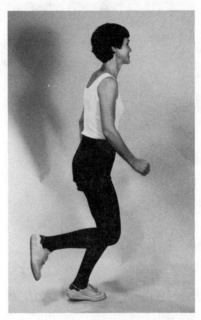

Figure 22B. Continue jogging in a circle

Figure 22C. Continue jogging in a circle

Figure 22D. Continue jogging in a circle

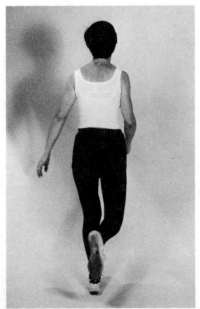

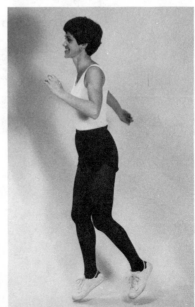

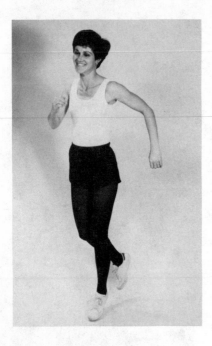

Figure 22E. Finish jogging in a circle

Jump: Both feet leave the floor together and return together, landing in the same place (Figure 23).

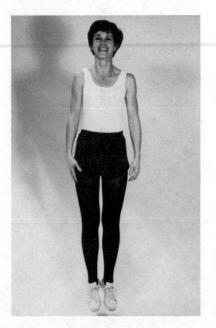

Figure 23. Jump

Hop: Standing on one foot, leave the floor and return, landing in the same place. Hops are done on either the left foot (Figure 24) or the right foot (Figure 25).

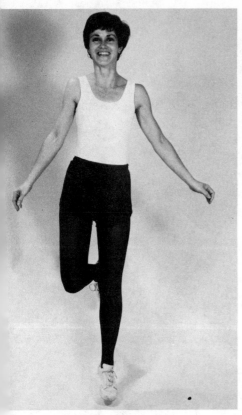

Figure 24. Hop left

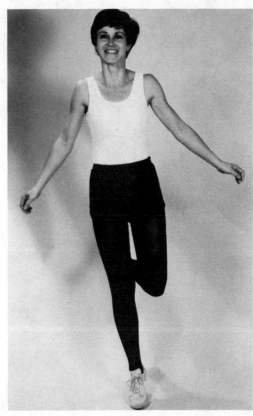

Figure 25. Hop right

Step Close Right: Step to the right with the right foot, step with left foot to meet right.

Step Close Left: Step to the left with the left foot, step with right foot to meet left.

Two Step: This is a three-movement motion like a quick 1-2-3 in place. Step right, step left, step right. (Figures 26A–26D). Or step left, step right, step left. Also called "Pony."

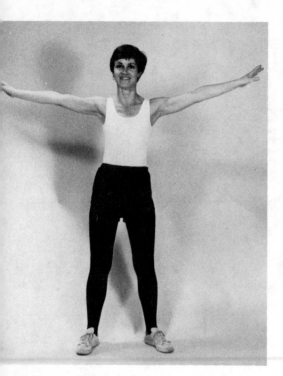

Figure 26A. Begin two-step pony

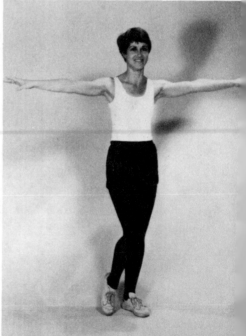

Figure 26B. Step left

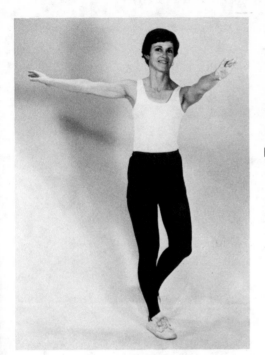

Figure 26C. Step right

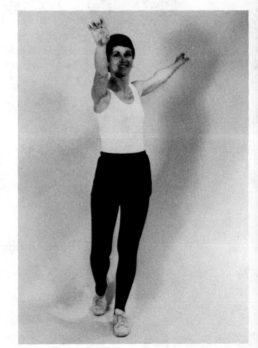

Figure 26D. Step left

Rock: With legs in a straddle position, hop from foot-to-foot, shifting body weight (Figures 27A and 27B).

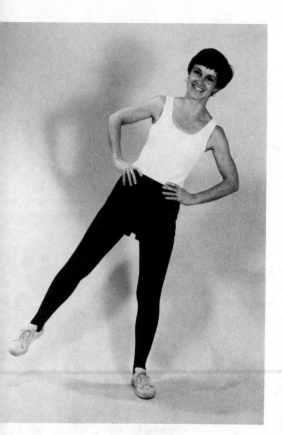

Figure 27A. Rock left

Figure 27B. Rock right

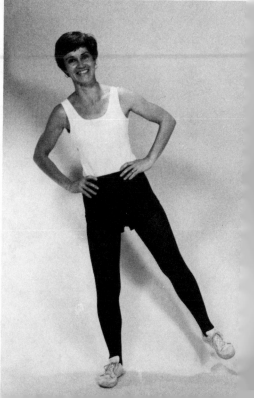

Rock Forward: With one leg slightly ahead of the other, hop from foot-to-foot forward and back, shifting body weight (Figure 28).

Figure 28. Rock forward

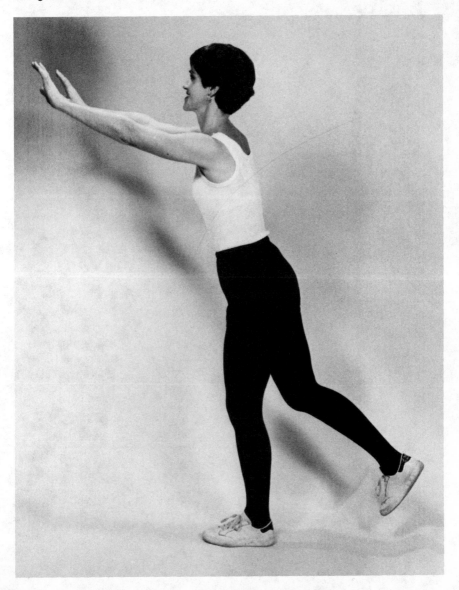

Slide Right: Step to the right with the right foot, slide left foot to meet right (Figures 29A and 29B).

Slide Left: Step to the left with the left foot, slide right foot to meet left.

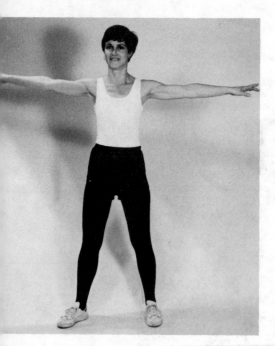

Figure 29A. Step right with right foot

Figure 29B. Slide left foot to meet right

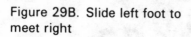

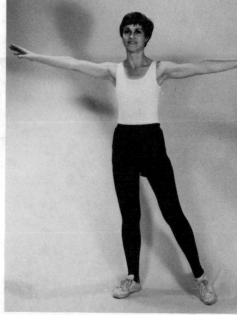

Pony: This is a three-movement motion like a quick 1-2-3 in place. Step right, step left, step right (see Figures 26A–26D). Or step left, step right, step left. Also called "Two-Step."

Step Kick Left: Step onto left foot while kicking right foot forward (Figures 30A and 30B).

Step Kick Right: Step onto the right foot while kicking left foot forward.

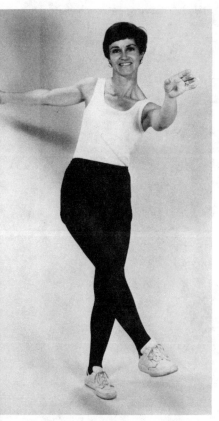 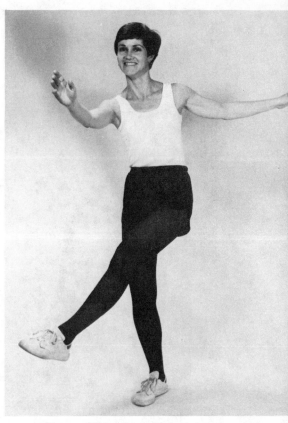

Figure 30A. Step kick left   Figure 30B. Step kick right

Swing Right: Begin with arms down at the sides and in front of the body. Keeping the body straight forward, swing both arms to the right, slightly higher than parallel to the floor (Figure 31).

Swing Left: Begin with arms down at the sides and in front of the body. Keeping the body straight forward, swing both arms to the left, slightly higher than parallel to the floor (Figure 32).

Figure 31. Swing right

Figure 32. Swing left

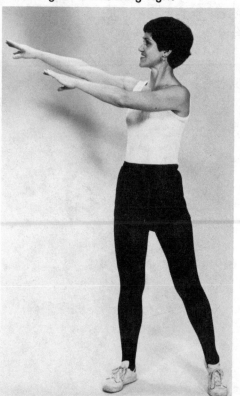 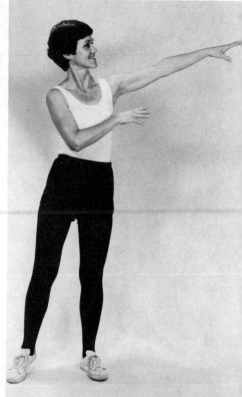

Hands to the Floor Left: Begin standing in a straddle position. Tuck your chin, bend from the waist and touch the floor to the left of the left foot with both hands (Figure 33).

Hands to the Floor Right: Begin standing in a straddle position. Tuck your chin, bend from the waist and touch the floor to the right of the right foot with both hands (Figure 34).

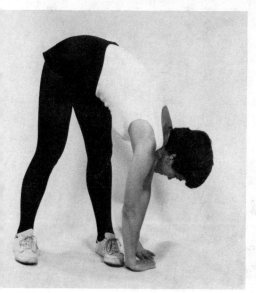

Figure 33. Palms to floor, left

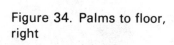

Figure 34. Palms to floor, right

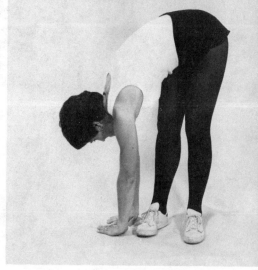

Hands to the Floor Center: Begin standing in a straddle position. Tuck your chin, bend from the waist and touch the floor between your feet (Figure 35).

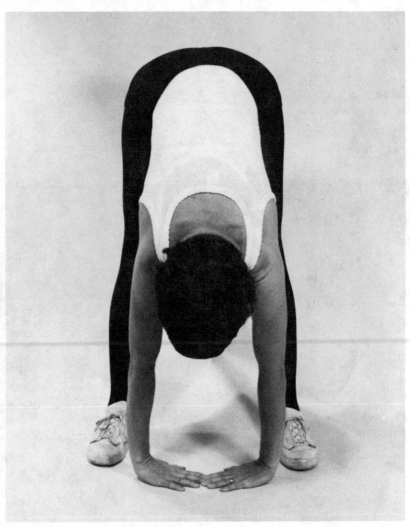

Figure 35. Palms to floor, center

Walk Out/Walk Back: Begin standing in a straddle position. Tuck your chin, bend from the waist until both hands touch the floor. Keeping heels on the floor, walk forward on hands. Hold. Walk back on hands, curl up and return to straddle position (Figures 36A and 36B).

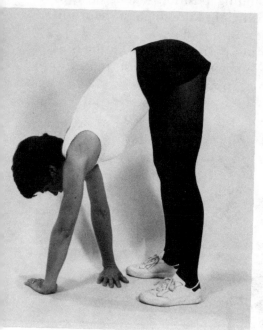

Figure 36A. Walk-out

Figure 36B. Walk-out further

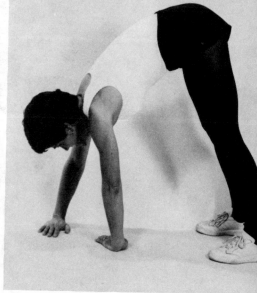

Knee Lift Right: In a standing position, hands on the hips or extended at shoulder level, lift right knee to chest, return (Figure 37).

Knee Lift Left: In a standing position, hands on the hips or extended at shoulder level, lift left knee to chest, return.

Double Knee Right: In a standing position, hands on hips or extended at shoulder level, lift right knee to chest, return to floor, lift right leg straight out, return to floor.

Double Knee Left: In a standing position, hands on the hips or extended at shoulder level, lift left knee to chest, return to floor, lift left leg straight out, return to floor.

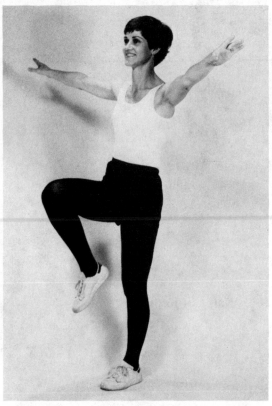

Figure 37. Knee-lift right

Chain Right: Step to the right with right foot, cross left leg over right (Figure 38A) and step on it, transferring weight (Figure 38B). Repeat for number of counts indicated.

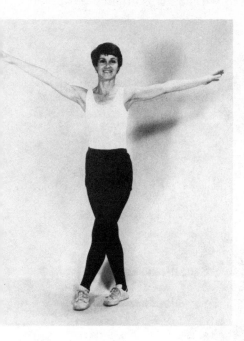

Figure 38A. Chain right—step to right with right foot, cross left leg over right

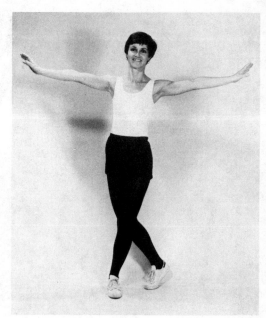

igure 38B. Transfer weight to left foot

Chain Left: Step to the left with left foot, cross right leg over left and step on it, transferring weight. Repeat for number of counts indicated (Figure 39).

Figure 39. Chain left—step to left with left foot, cross right leg over left, and transfer weight

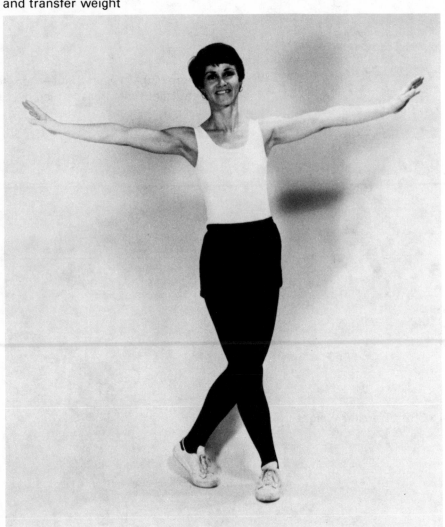

Floor Sweep Left: Start in straddle position with arms overhead (Figure 40A). Bend from the waist turning left while arms separate (Figure 40B) and circle down toward the floor (Figure 40C). Continue circle as you return (Figure 40D) to starting position.

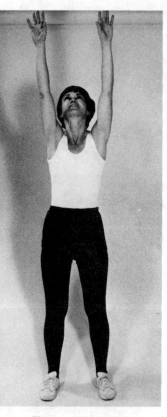

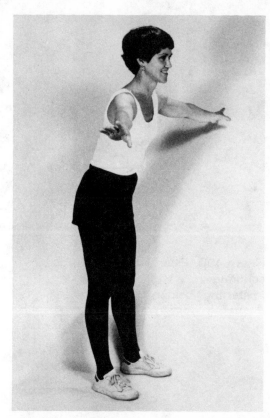

Figure 40A. Floor sweep—start in straddle position, reach high over head

Figure 40B. Floor sweep—bend from waist to left while arms separate

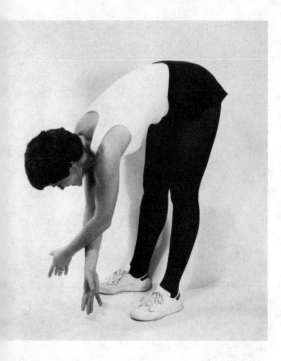

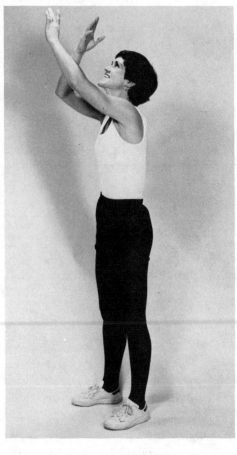

Figure 40C. Floor sweep—
circle down toward floor

Figure 40D. Floor sweep—
continue circle while returning
to starting position

Floor Sweep Right: Start in straddle position with arms overhead. Bend from the waist turning right while arms separate and circle down toward the floor. Continue circle as you return to starting position.

Floor Sweep Center: Start in straddle position with arms overhead. Bend from the waist while arms separate and circle down toward the floor. Continue arm circle as you return to starting position.

Trunk Circle Left: Start in straddle position with arms overhead. Bend from the waist while arms separate and circle down to the floor (Figure 41A). Moving both arms together, swing arms up left side (Figure 41B), overhead (Figure 41C), down the right side (Figure 41D), and back down to the floor in a sweeping motion (Figure 41E). Either repeat two-arm circle or return to starting position.

Figure 41A. Trunk circle—bend from waist while arms separate

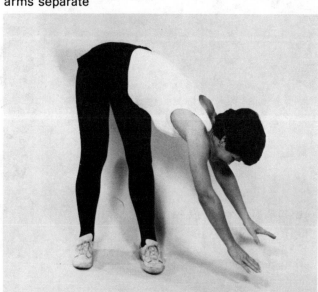

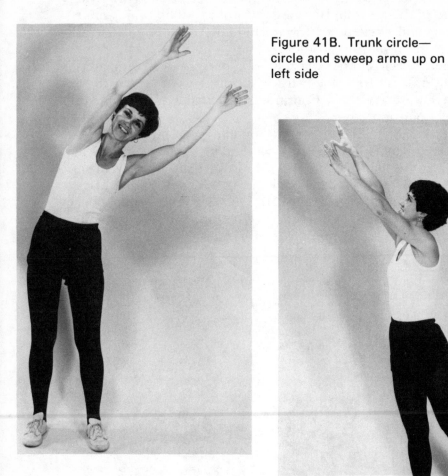

Figure 41B. Trunk circle—circle and sweep arms up on left side

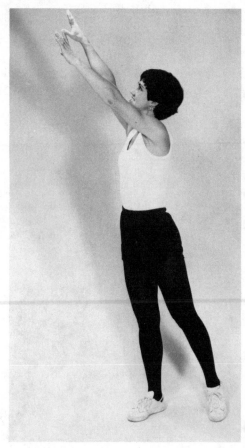

Figure 41C. Trunk circle—swing overhead . . .

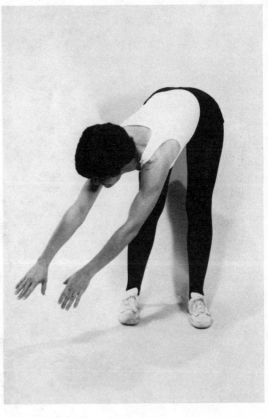

Figure 41D. and down right side

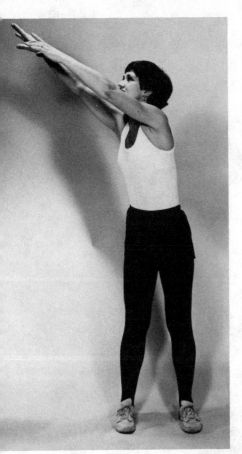

Figure 41E. Back down to the floor in a sweeping motion

Trunk Circle Right: Start in straddle position with arms overhead. Bend from the waist while arms separate and circle down to the floor. Moving both arms together, swing arms up right side, overhead, down the left side and back to the floor in a sweeping motion. Either repeat two-arm circle or return to starting position.

Half-Knee Bend: In a standing position with feet together and legs straight, bend knees to about a 45-degree angle (Figure 42). Return to starting position.

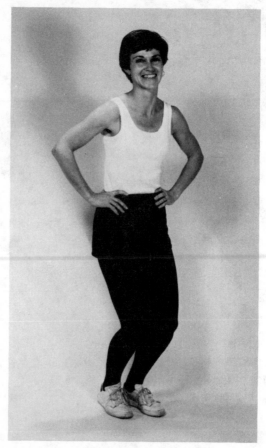

Figure 42. Half-knee bend

Twist: Stand with feet on the floor, body straight. Turn lower body to the left and upper body to the right (Figure 43). Repeat in opposite direction.

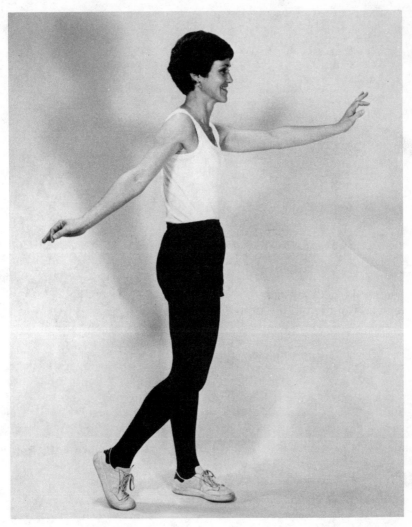

Figure 43. Twist right

Crazy Kick Right: Stand on left foot, extend right leg to the right side (Figure 44A), return (Figure 44B), extend (Figure 44C), return.

Crazy Kick Left: Stand on right foot, extend left leg to the left side, return, extend, return.

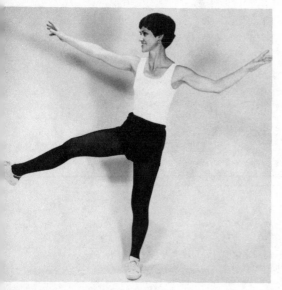

Figure 44A. Crazy kick—
extend right leg to the right

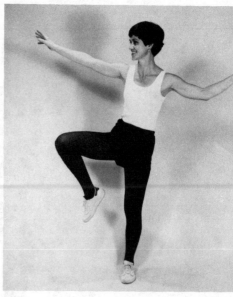

Figure 44B. Return . . .

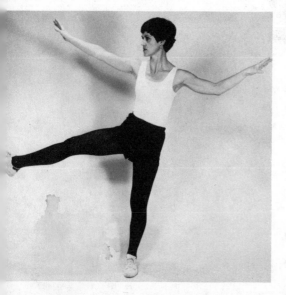

Figure 44C. and extend

Lunge Left: Stand in straddle position. Shift weight to the left while bending left knee (Figure 45). Return to starting position.

Lunge Right: Stand in straddle position. Shift weight to the right while bending right knee. Return to starting position.

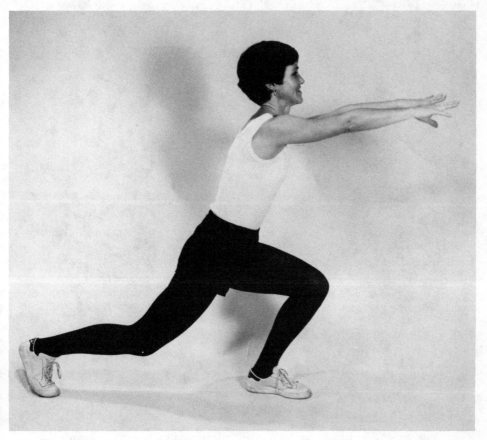

Figure 45. Lunge left

Lunge Forward: Stand in straddle position, except position legs one ahead of the other. Shift weight to the right while bending right knee. Arms may be extended forward (Figure 46A) or down in front with hands resting on knees (Figure 46B). Return to starting position.

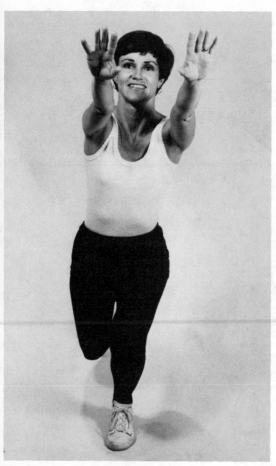

Figure 46A. Lunge forward, arms extended

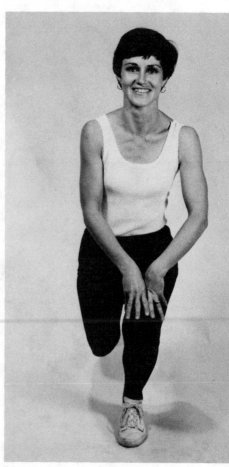

Figure 46B. Lunge forward, hands on knees

Push-Up: Face-down on the floor, resting on bent-knees and hands in diamond-shape (see Figure 12) and keeping the back straight, raise and lower your body with the arms. (See Chapter 5 for cautions in doing this exercise.)

Reverse Push-Up: Sitting on the floor with legs extended and upper body resting on hands, lift the body up, hold, return (Figure 47).

Swing: Pony or two-step in place while arms move or swing side-to-side.

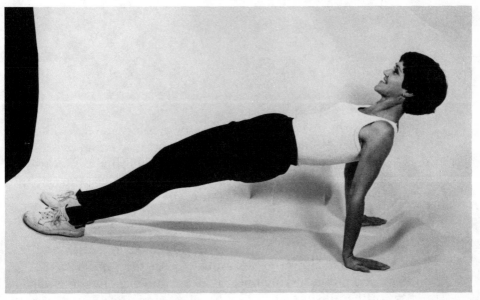

Figure 47. Reverse push-up

8
Warming Up

A good warm-up is essential to any aerobic activity. The series of exercises alerts your heart to the upcoming work, raises your body temperature, and loosens and stretches muscles to prevent injury. Warming up to music is a pleasant way to get the blood flowing, in addition to getting your mind and body into the "swing of things."

To make it easier for you to familiarize yourself with matching routines to music, we will suggest song titles and recording artists. However, any music with the same beat or tempo is acceptable. Remember, match your movements with the beat of the music.

Your warm-up program is made up of four routines: "Alley Cat," "And the Beat Goes On," "The Main Event" (short version), and "Still the Same."

Begin by walking around the room for about sixty seconds, just to get yourself moving. Then:

ALLEY CAT
Artist: Bent Fabric
Time: 2:23

Wait for short introduction.

Touch the floor with both hands
Touch hips with hands
Reach up with both hands overhead
Touch hips

Touch the floor
Touch hips
Reach up
Touch hips

Touch floor
Touch hips
Reach up
Touch hips

Touch floor
Touch hips
Reach up
Touch hips

Touch outside your left foot with both hands
Touch hips
Reach up
Touch hips

Touch outside your right foot with both hands
Touch hips
Reach up
Touch hips

Touch outside your left foot with both hands
Touch hips
Reach up
Touch hips

Touch outside your right foot with both hands
Touch hips
Reach up
Touch hips

Raise both shoulders up and down 8 times

Raise right shoulder up and down 4 times

Raise left shoulder up and down 4 times

Rotate shoulders forward 4 times

Rotate shoulders backward 4 times

(extend arms at shoulder level)
Rotate arms forward (palms up) 4 times

Rotate arms backward 4 times

Alternate arm rotation 8 times

(extend arms at shoulder level)
Reach left—hold 4 counts

Reach right—hold 4 counts

Reach left—hold 4 counts

Right right—hold 4 counts

(arms extended at shoulder level)
Lunge Left—hold 4 counts

Lunge right—hold 4 counts

Lunge left—hold 4 counts

Lunge right—hold 4 counts

Touch floor
Touch hips
Reach up
Touch hips

Touch floor
Touch hips

Reach up
Touch hips

Touch floor
Touch hips
Reach up
Touch hips

Touch floor
Touch hips
Reach up
Touch hips

Touch outside left foot with both hands
Touch hips
Reach up
Touch hips

Touch outside right foot with both hands
Touch hips
Reach up
Touch hips

Touch outside left foot with both hands
Touch hips
Reach up
Touch hips

Touch outside right foot with both hands
Touch hips
Reach up
Touch hips

AND THE BEAT GOES ON
Artist: The Whispers
Time: 3:25

Move right arm across body—left to right
Move left arm across body—right to left

Toe touch with right foot—2 front, 2 back, 1 front, 1 back, 1
    side (bring left foot to right)
Toe touch with left foot—2 front, 2 back, 1 front, 1 back, 1
    side (bring right foot to left)
Toe touch with right foot—2 front, 2 back, 1 front, 1 back, 1
    side (bring left foot to right)
Toe touch with left foot—2 front, 2 back, 1 front, 1 back, 1
    side (bring right foot to left)

Chain right—1, 2, 3, kick
Chain left—1, 2, 3, kick
Chain right
Chain left
Chain right
Chain left
Chain right
Chain left

Toe touch with right foot—2 front, 2 back, 1 front, 1 back, 1
    side (bring left foot to right)
Toe touch with left foot—2 front, 2 back, 1 front, 1 back, 1
    side (bring right foot to left)
Toe touch with right foot—2 front, 2 back, 1 front, 1 back, 1
    side (bring left foot to right)
Toe touch with left foot—2 front, 2 back, 1 front, 1 back, 1
    side (bring right foot to left)
Turn to the right—clap 2
Turn to the left—clap 2
Turn to the right—clap 2
Turn left—clap 2
Turn right—clap 2
Turn left—clap 2
Turn right—clap 2
Turn left—clap 2

Toe touches with right foot
Toe touches with left foot
Toe touches with right foot
Toe touches with left foot
Hip swivel to right (step right, bring left to meet right)—4
    times
Hip swivel to left (step left, bring right to meet left)—4 times
Hip swivel to right
Hip swivel to left

Toe touches with right foot
Toe touches with left foot
Toe touches with right foot
Toe touches with left foot

Chain right
Chain left
Chain right
Chain left
Chain right
Chain left
Chain right
Chain left

Toe touches with right foot
Toe touches with left foot
Toe touches with right foot
Toe touches with left foot

Turn to the right—clap 2
Turn to the left—clap 2
Turn right—clap 2
Turn left—clap 2
Turn right—clap 2
Turn left—clap 2
Turn right—clap 2
Turn left—clap 2

Toe touches with right foot
Toe touches with left foot
Toe touches with right foot
Toe touches with left foot

Hip swivel to right—4 times
Hip swivel to left—4 times
Hip swivel to right—4 times
Hip swivel to left—4 times

THE MAIN EVENT (short version)
Artist: Barbra Streisand
Time: 4:51

Floor sweep center—2 times
Trunk circle left—2 times
Trunk circle right—2 times

Half-knee bends to right—8
Half-knee bends to left—8
Half-knee bends right—4
Half-knee bends left—4
Half-knee bends right—2
Half-knee bends left—2
Half-knee bends right—2
Half-knee bends left—2

Hip to the right side—8
Hip to the left side—8
Hip to the right—4
Hip to the left—4
Hip to the right—2
Hip to the left—2
Hip to the right—2
Hip to the left—2

Twist facing left—8
Twist facing right—8
Twist left—4
Twist right—4
Twist left—2
Twist right—2
Twist left—2
Twist right—2

Shadow box left—8
Shadow box right—8
Shadow box left—4
Shadow box right—4
Shadow box left—2
Shadow box right—2
Shadow box left—2
Shadow box right—2

Floor sweep and stretch—8 counts
Floor sweep and stretch—8 counts

Start at the beginning and repeat throughout until record ends.

STILL THE SAME
Artist: Bob Seger
Time: 3:20

Hands to the floor on the left side
Reach up—center
Hands to the floor—right
Reach up—center

Hands to floor—left
Reach up—center
Hands to floor—right
Reach up—center

Hands to floor—left
Reach up—center
Hands to floor—right
Reach up—center

Hands to floor—left
Reach up—center
Hands to floor—right
Reach up—center

Hands to floor—left
Reach up—center
Hands to floor—right
Reach up—center

Hands to floor—left
Reach up—center
Hands to floor—right
Reach up—center

Hands to floor—left
Reach up—center
Hands to floor—right
Reach up—center

Hands to floor—left
Reach up—center
Hands to floor—right
Reach up—center

Walk out—4 counts
Flex hips toward the floor
Flex hips toward the ceiling
Hips to floor
Hips to ceiling
Hips to floor
Hips to ceiling
Hips to floor
Hips to ceiling
Walk back—4 counts

Start at the beginning and repeat throughout until record ends.

Caution

1. Be sure to round your back when reaching for the floor and going back up.
2. Raise and lower your hips to your own degree of flexibility.

9
Aerobic Dance Routines

Now that you're nice and warmed up, go right into the aerobic routines. Do not take time out to cool off; once you are working, it is important to continue.

During the routines, if you are out of breath or simply can't keep step, slow down and, perhaps, do every other beat. Do not stop abruptly. If you prefer a shorter aerobic activity, cut from these nine routines, then go into the cool-downs. Remember, though, with continued activity, your entire body, including the muscles and the cardiovascular system, will become stronger and the routines easier.

As with the warm-up numbers, we offer suggested music and recording artists. Again, if you can't find or don't like a particular number, use an alternate that offers the same tempo. Here are the recordings we use: "Dancing Bumble Bee," "Tusk," "Rock Around the Clock," "Volcano," "The Entertainer," "Mame," "Fame," "Hound Dog," and "Rise."

DANCING BUMBLE BEE
Artist: Neil Diamond
Time: 4:53

Squat (straight back)—8 times

Reach right
Reach left
Reach right
Reach left
Reach right
Reach left
Reach right
Reach left

Jog circle—8 counts

Jumping Jacks—8 times

Start at the beginning and repeat throughout until record ends.

Take your pulse

TUSK
Artist: Fleetwood Mac
Time: 3:36

Pony right
Pony left
Pony right
Pony left
Pony right
Pony left
Pony right
Pony left

Rock—8 times

Rock forward—8 times

Step kick—8 times

Squat—8 times

Slide right—4 times
Slide left—4 times

Swing—8 times

Start at the beginning and repeat throughout until record ends.

Take your pulse; keep walking or moving your legs as you do.

ROCK AROUND THE CLOCK
Artist: Bill Haley and The Comets
Time: 2:08

Twist—32

Step kick—4
Jog forward—8
Step kick in circle right—4
Step kick in circle left—4
Twist—16

Step kick—4
Jog backward—8

Step kick in circle—4
Change directions—4
Twist—16

Rock and kick (begin to left)—12

Step kick—4
Jog forward—8
Step kick in circle—4
Change directions—4
Twist—16

Step kick—4
Jog backward—8
Step kick in circle—4
Change directions—4
Twist—16

Crazy kick—12
Step kick—4
Jog forward—8
Step kick—4
Jog forward—8
Step kick in circle—4
Change directions—4
Twist to end of music

Take your pulse; keep walking or moving your legs as you do.

VOLCANO
Artist: Jimmy Buffett
Time: 3:37

Knee lift right
Knee lift left

Jump jump

Knee lift right
Knee lift left

Jump jump

Knee lift right
Knee lift left

Jump jump

Knee lift right
Knee lift left

Jump jump

Double knee—6
1 2 3 4 up on toes and down—3

Chain right 3 and kick left
Chain left 3 and kick right

Knee lift left
Knee lift right
Jump jump

Chain right 3 and kick left
Chain left 3 and kick right

Knee lift left
Knee lift right
Jump jump

Chain right 3 and kick left
Chain left 3 and kick right

Knee lift left
Knee lift right
Jump jump

Chain right 3 and kick left
Chain left 3 and kick right

Knee lift left
Knee lift right
Jump jump

Double knee—6
1 2 3 4 up on toes and down—4

Kick forward—4

Jog circle—4

Jump jump

Kick forward—4

Jog circle—4

Jump jump

Kick forward—4

Jog circle—4

Jump jump

Kick forward—4

Jog circle—4

Jump jump

Double knee—6
1 2 3 4 up on toes and down—4

Double knee—6
1 2 3 4 up on toes and down—4

Run forward—4
Run back—4
Jog—4
Jump jump

Run forward—4
Run back—4
Jog—4
Jump jump

Run forward—4
Run back—4
Jog—4
Jump jump

Run forward—4
Run back—4
Jog—4
Jump jump

Double knee—6
1 2 3 4 up on toes and down

Double knee—6
1 2 3 4 up on toes and down

Chain right 3, kick left
Chain left 3, kick right
Knee lift left
Knee lift right
Jump jump

Chain right 3, kick left
Chain left 3, kick right
Knee lift left
Knee lift right
Jump jump

Kick forward—4
Jog circle—4
Jump jump

Kick forward—4
Jog circle—4
Jump jump

Run forward—4
Run back—4
Jog—4

Jump jump

Run forward—4
Run back—4
Jog—4

Jump jump

Double knee—6
1 2 3 4 up on toes and down—4

Double knee—6
1 2 3 4 up on toes and down—4

Take your pulse; be sure to keep walking or moving your legs
as you do.

THE ENTERTAINER
(any version)

Jump (legs apart, apart, together)—3

Touch floor with right knee and jump up

*Hop on right foot—8
Jog—8

Hop on left foot—8
Jog—8

Hop on right foot—8
Jog—8

Hop on left foot—8
Jog—8

Step close to right—4
Two-step right-left—2
Rock—3 (slight hesitation)
Step close to left—4
Two-step right-left—2
Rock—4

Step close to right—4
Two-step right-left—2
Rock—3 (slight hesitation)
Step close to left—4
Two-step right-left—2
Rock—4

Right foot heel-toe—4
Slide right—4
Left foot heel-toe—4
Slide left—4

Right foot heel-toe—4
Slide right—4
Left foot heel-toe—4
Slide left—4

Go back to asterisk (*) and complete entire routine.

Rock—8
Rock forward (begin forward right)—8
Rock—7 (slight hesitation)
Rock forward—7 (slight hesitation)

Jump—3
Touch floor with right knee and jump up

Hop right foot—8
Jog—8

Hop left foot—8
Jog—8

Hop right foot—8
Jog—8

Hop left foot—8
Jog—8

Take your pulse; keep walking or moving your legs as you do.

MAME
Artist: Herb Alpert
Time: 2:08

Step right, chain right—8
Rock—8
Cross left, chain left—8
Rock—8
Step kick (begin step right, kick left)—8
Forward (begin right)—4
Back (begin left)—4
Forward (begin right)—4
Back (begin left)—4

Step right, chain right—8
Rock—8
Cross left, chain left—8
Rock—8
Step kick (begin step right, kick left)—8
Forward (begin right)—4
Back (begin left)—4
Forward (begin right)—4
Back (begin left)—4

Step kick (begin step right, kick left)—4
Break (jump back slightly)—4

Step right, chain right—8
Rock—8
Cross left and chain left—8
Rock—8
Step kick (begin right, kick left)—8
Forward (begin right)—4
Back (begin left)—4
Forward (begin right)—4
Back (begin left)—4

Step right, chain right—8
Rock—8
Cross left and chain left—8
Rock—8
Step kick (begin right, kick left)—8
Forward (begin right)—4
Back (begin left)—4
Forward (begin right)—4
Back (begin left)—4

Step right, chain right—8
Rock—8
Cross left, chain left—8
Rock—8
Step kick (begin right, kick left)—8
Forward (begin right)—4

Back (begin left)—4
Forward (begin right)—4
Back (begin left)—4

Forward—4
Back—4
Forward—4
Back—4

Step kick (begin right, kick left)—4
Break (jump back slightly)—4

Take your pulse; keep moving or walking as you do.

FAME
Artist: Irene Cara
Time: 3:48

Step back left right left
Clap—2
Step forward right left right
Clap—2

Step back left right left
Clap—2
Step forward right left right
Clap—2

1 2 3 Pony while turning side to side—8
(begin with right foot facing right, then with left foot facing
    left)

Step back left right left
Clap—2
Step forward right left right
Clap—2

Step back left right left
Clap—2
Step forward right left right
Clap—2

1 2 3 Pony (begin with right foot)—8

Step back left right left
Clap—2
Step forward right left right
Clap—2

Step back left right left
Clap—2
Step forward right left right
Clap—2

1 2 and 1 2 3 Pony while moving side-to-side—8
(begin with right foot to right then left foot to right then
     quick-step right, left, right)

Repeat 1 2 and 1 2 3 Pony to left—8

Repeat entire routine until music ends.

Take your pulse; keep walking or moving your legs as you do.

HOUND DOG
Artist: Elvis Presley
Time: 2:13

Crazy kick right—4
Crazy kick left—4
Crazy kick right—2
Crazy kick left—2
Crazy kick—1 right, 1 left, 1 right, 1 left

Crazy kick right—4
Crazy kick left—4
Crazy kick right—2
Crazy kick left—2
Crazy kick—1 right, 1 left, 1 right, 1 left

Crazy kick right—4
Crazy kick left—4
Crazy kick right—2
Crazy kick left—2
Crazy kick—1 right, 1 left, 1 right, 1 left

Twist right—4
Twist left—4
Twist right—4
Twist left—4
Twist in circle—8

Crazy kick right—4
Crazy kick left—4
Crazy kick right—2
Crazy kick left—2
Crazy kick—1 right, 1 left, 1 right, 1 left

Twist right—4
Twist left—4
Twist right—4
Twist left—4
Twist in circle—8

Crazy kick right—4
Crazy kick left—4
Crazy kick right—2
Crazy kick left—2
Crazy kick—1 right, 1 left, 1 right, 1 left

Crazy kick right—4
Crazy kick left—4
Crazy kick right—2
Crazy kick left—2
Crazy kick—1 right, 1 left, 1 right, 1 left

Take your pulse; keep walking or moving your legs as you do.

RISE
Artist: Herb Alpert
Time: 3:45

Starting position: Sit on floor, legs extended, body resting on both arms in comfortable position.

Bicycle—8
Bicycle to left—8
Bicycle center—8
Bicycle to right—8

Break 4 times—feet touch (8 counts) floor touch on 4 counts
(touch and hold)

Repeat to end of record.

Take your pulse. Remember to keep walking. Walk around the
room for 60 seconds. Take your pulse again. This time it
should be 120 beats—20 in your 10-second count—or less.

If your pulse has not dropped to 120 or less, continue
walking another 60 seconds or until your heart rate has come
down.

When your heart is 120 or less, go on to the Cool-Downs.

10
Cool-Downs

Remember, all aerobic activities are three-phase programs—warm-ups, aerobics and cool-downs. The three share equal importance. If you must trim something, cut down on the aerobics sections—but not less than twelve minutes in duration. Never skip or slight either the warm-ups or cool-downs.

Cool-downs have two important functions. First, they keep the muscles stretched out until they are cool or have returned to normal body temperature. Second, the continued but slower activity prevents the blood from pooling in the lower leg.

We suggest that cool-downs not be done to music, because they should be done at your own speed. When you have music in the background, you tend to be locked into a pace or a beat that can be either too fast or too slow to suit you and your particular needs.

Immediately after you have finished your last aerobic routine and have checked your pulse, walk for sixty seconds. Check your pulse again. Remember, a healthy heart will drop in that minute to 120 beats or below, then level off.

If, initially, your pulse is faster than twenty beats in the ten-second count, walk a little longer. Once you are at 120 or less, begin your stretches and cool-downs. If you began working wearing a warm-up jacket, now is the time to put it back on.

Pick up your cobra and, while continuing to walk, stretch it:

At hip level—4 times
At chest level—4
Up and slightly forward—4
At chest—4

At hip—4
At chest—4
Up and slightly forward—4
At chest—4

From your left shoulder (Figure 48)—4
From your right shoulder—4
From your left shoulder—4
From your right shoulder—4

Forward from your forehead, left hand—4
Forward from your forehead, right hand—4
Forward from your forehead, left hand—4
Forward from your forehead, right hand—4

Forward from hip level, left hand—4
Forward from hip level, right hand—4
Forward from hip, left hand—4
Forward from hip, right hand—4

From left shoulder—4
From right shoulder—4
From left shoulder—4
From right shoulder—4

Forward from forehead, left hand—4
Forward from forehead, right hand—4
Forward from forehead, left hand—4
Forward from forehead, right hand—4

From hip, left hand—4
From hip, right hand—4
From hip, left hand—4
From hip, right hand—4

At hip level—4
At chest level—4

Lay the cobra down. Put your feet together, flat on the floor. Maintaining that position,
    Rotate your thighs to the outside
    Tighten your abdominal muscles
    Tighten your buttocks muscles
    Squeeze buttocks muscles together
    Tuck buttocks muscles under.
Concentrate and continue to hold everything from the waist down just as tight as you can for 15 seconds.
Make sure you are breathing!
Relax and shake your legs out.
Now, get down on the floor for these cool-down and strength-flexibility exercises:

1. Reverse push-up. Sit on the floor with your legs straight out in front as you lean back on your arms. Raise your body slowly so all of your weight is on your hands and your feet (see Figure 47). Slowly and with control, lower yourself to starting position. Do 10 Reverse Push-Ups.
Shake your legs out and shrug your shoulders a few times to loosen them up.
2. Grab your toes. Sit on the floor with your legs straight out in front as you lean forward and grab your toes. Get a good hold on them and do not worry about bent knees. Pull your toes toward you as you try to extend them toward the opposite wall (Figure 48). Hold that stretch. Make sure you are breathing!
Relax and shake your arms and legs out.

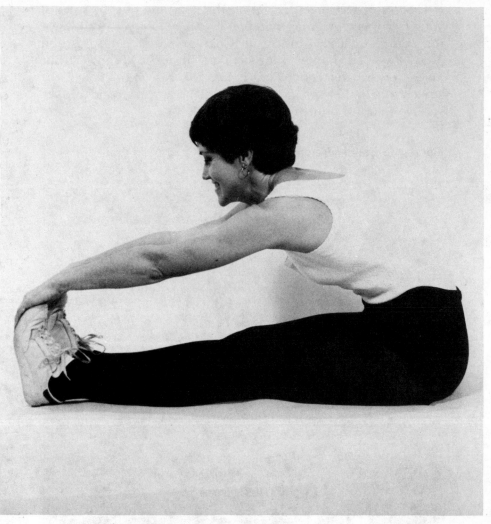

Figure 48. Toe stretch

3. **Grab your ankles.** Sit on the floor with your legs straight out in front and lean forward to grab your ankles. *Slowly* pull your upper body toward your legs. *Do not bounce.* Feel a good stretch? Hold it for at least ten seconds. Make sure you are breathing.

4. Soles of feet together. Sit on the floor and put the soles of your feet together. Your hands can either hold your ankles or they can be placed behind you. Changing your hand position every day or so changes your stretch a little. Slowly lower your knees toward the floor (Figure 49). *Do not bounce.* Feel the stretch and hold your position for at least ten seconds. Make sure you do not hold your breath.

Figure 49. Tailor stretch

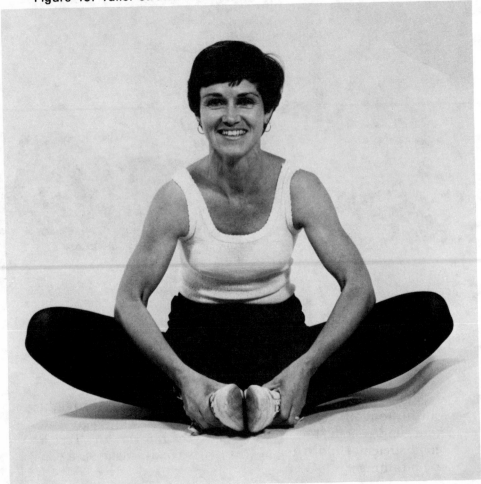

5. Side leg raises. Lie down on your left side. Keep your body in a straight line. Your head is positioned on an outstretched arm above your head. Try to keep your body straight throughout the exercise and try to keep your leg lifting up rather than to the front.

Do not worry about how high your leg is; lift until you feel a good stretch.

Remember, you work muscles on the way down as well as on the way up, so tighten your leg muscles and move up and down slowly and with control.

a. Bring your right foot to your left knee (Figure 50).

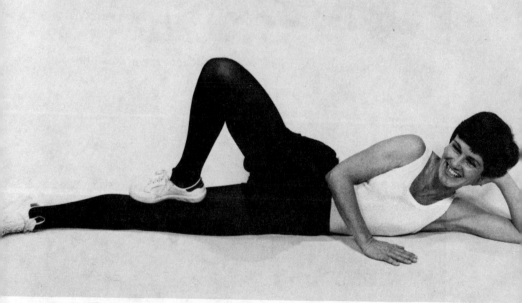

Figure 50. Right foot to left knee

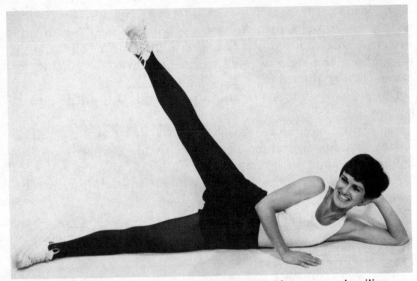

Figure 51. Single side leg raise. Raise right foot toward ceiling

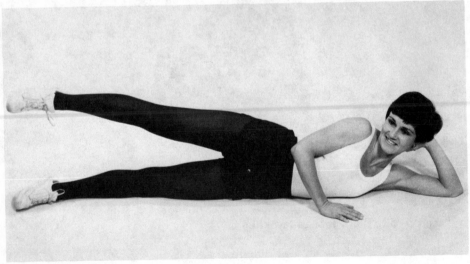

Figure 52. Lower right leg to left leg

Straighten your right leg up toward the ceiling (Figure 51). Lower right leg to left leg (Figure 52). Do this exercise 8 times.

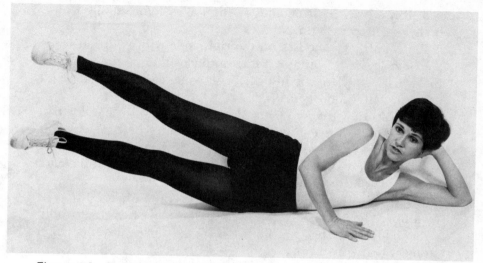

Figure 53. Bring left leg to meet right

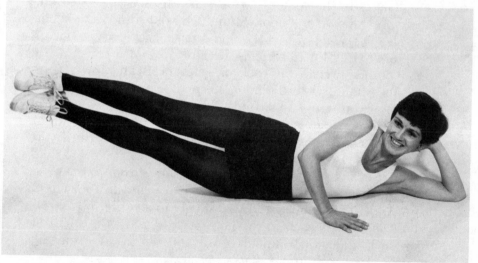

Figure 54. Lower both legs together

b. Keeping your right leg straight, raise it slowly as high as is comfortable. Lower to your left leg. Repeat 8 times.

c. Raise your right leg. Bring your left leg up (Figure 53) until both legs meet (Figure 54). Lower both legs together. Repeat 8 times.

d. Raise both legs together as high as is comfortable. Lower both legs. Repeat 8 times.

Repeat all leg exercises on the right side with your left leg.

These leg raises are good for toning of thighs, the hips and the waist area. Do not strain! Raise your legs until you feel a good stretch, hold, then lower.

6. Push-ups. Lie on your stomach with your hands in a diamond shape (see Figure 12) under your chest. With your knees bent (see Figure 13), raise and lower your body with your arms and shoulders. Take your time. Stop if you have to, but try to continue on and do 10 push-ups.

Keep your body as straight as you can. Make sure you breathe. When you have enough abdominal strength to hold your body straight (see Figure 14), you may advance to a straight body push-up.

Make sure you feel no back discomfort. You do *not* want to injure your back!

7. Back stretch. Assume your push-up starting position. Keep your hips on the floor. Straighten your arms as much as possible. Put your head back and stretch back *only as far as feels good*. Hold for 10 seconds. Breathe!

8. Another stretch. Sit back on your heels and lower your head and shoulders to the floor. Keep your arms stretched out in front of you. Hold 10 seconds. Breathe.

9. Backward stretch. Raise up to a kneeling position. Keeping your body straight, lean slowly backwards until you feel a stretch. Do not bounce! Relax.

10. Sit-ups. Lie down on your back and bend your knees. Raise your head off the floor and tuck your chin to your chest. Keep your back rounded and curl slowly to a sitting position.

Lower yourself back to the floor starting with the small of your back and slowly uncurl until you are in your starting position. Repeat 10 times.

Never jerk up! Always round your back.

If you cannot come to a sitting position, bring your head and shoulders off the floor and hold until your abdominal muscles start to quiver, then lower slowly back to floor.

Take your time. Work at your own speed. And make sure you are breathing.

11. Leg extensions. Lie on your back with your knees to your chest and your head up off the floor. Your hands need to be placed at the small of your back to monitor the amount of back-arch when your legs are extended. If, when you extend your legs, your back arches, you *must* extend your legs higher off the floor to keep from straining your back.

Extend legs slowly and then tuck your knees back to your chest. Repeat 10 times.

Put your feet down, straighten your legs. Take a deep breath and exhale slowly. Again and exhale slowly.

12. Legs up. Support the small of your back with your hands and raise your legs up toward the ceiling. Hold your position about 15 seconds.

Lower your knees to your forehead. Point your toes toward the ceiling and hold 15 seconds.

Extend your legs out over your head so your toes are on the floor. Walk out as far as you can. Try to tuck your chin into the base of your neck. Hold 15 seconds.

Support your back with your hands and raise your legs up again. Hold 15 seconds.

13. Neck stretches. Lower your knees to your forehead. Cross one leg over the other. Curl up to a sitting position. Curl over, head toward the floor and stretch. Hold 10 seconds.

Raise your head slowly. Put your hands on the floor behind you and stretch back. Hold 10 seconds.

Raise your head. Slowly turn and look over your left shoulder as far as possible. Hold 10 seconds.

Look straight ahead. Slowly turn and look over your right shoulder as far as possible. Hold 10 seconds.

Lower your head forward and rotate your head in a circle to the left. Slowly. Go as far in every direction as you can. When you complete a rotation, change directions and rotate slowly to the right.

Drop your head forward and relax.

Raise your head just enough to enable yourself to inhale slowly and deeply. Hold it 5 seconds and exhale slowly. Repeat 3 times.

You can close your eyes during the head rotations and deep breathing if this helps you to relax.

Congratulations! You have just completed your first aerobic dance routine. We hope this is the beginning of a new way of life for you.

Remember, a better feeling about yourself comes through better health that results from better physical fitness.

If you will now dedicate yourself to an aerobic routine a minimum of three times a week for three weeks, you will begin to notice a remarkable change in yourself—mentally as well as physically—and the whole world will take on new meaning.

Welcome to the world of feeling good!

Index

A

Aerobic exercise, 4
Aerobic dance, 9
   routines, 72–85
Aging, 7
"Alley Cat," 63–64
"And the Beat Goes On,"
   65–68

B

Back, avoiding strain, 26
Back stretch, 96
Backward stretch, 96
Bicycle, to left, 28
   to right, 28
Bra, picking correct, 12

C

Calf, cramps in, 25
Cardiovascular system, 2–3
Chain left, 50
   right, 49
Clothing, 11–15
Cobra, 19, 87–88
Cool-down, 25
   routines, 86–96
Crazy kick left, 58
   right, 58
Cureton, Thomas K., 2

D

"Dancing Bumble Bee," 73
Double knee left, 48
   right, 48

E

"Entertainer, The," 79–80

F

"Fame," 82–83
Fitness, 5
Floor sweeps, center, 53
  left, 51
  right, 53

G

Grab your ankles, 89
Grab your toes, 88

H

Half knee bend, 56
Hands to floor center, 46
  left, 45
  right, 45
Heart disease, 2
Heart rate, 18
Hop, 37
"Hound Dog," 83–84

J

Jog circle, 35
Jump, 36
Jumping Jack, 30

K

Keelor, Dr. Richard, 2

Knee lift left, 48
  right, 48

L

Leg extensions, 97
Legs up, 97
Lunge forward, 61
  left, 59
  right, 59

M

"Main Event, The," 68–69
"Mame," 80–82
Muscles, stretching, 27
Myers, Clayton R., 5

N

Neck stretches, 95

P

Pony, 43
President's Council on
  Physical Fitness, 2
Pulse rate, 17, 87
Push-ups, 22–23, 61, 96

R

Reach left, 32
  right, 32
Reach up, 34
Reverse push-up, 61, 88
"Rise," 84–85

"Rock around the Clock,"
74–75
Rock, 40
  forward, 41

S

Shoes, 12–14
Side leg raises, 91–94
Sit-ups, 27, 96
Slide left, 42
  right, 42
Soles of feet together, 90
Squat, 32
Step close left, 37
  right, 37
Step kick left, 43
  right, 43
"Still the Same," 69–71
Straddle, 28
Straddle Jump, 30
Stress, 6
Swing, 61
  left, 44
  right, 44

T

Talk test, 19
Trunk circle left, 53
  right, 56
"Tusk," 73–74
Twist, 57
Two-step, 38

U

Upper arm toning, 19

V

"Volcano," 75–78

W

Walk out/walk back, 47
Warm-up, 24
  routines, 62–71
Weight gain, 10
  loss, 9